I0440671

Paleo Diet Side Effects?

By M. Usman

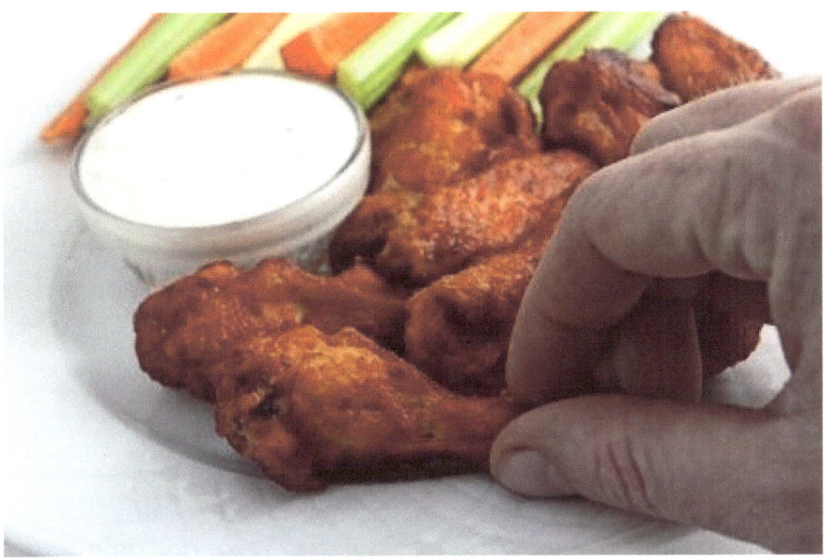

Health Learning Series

Mendon Cottage Books

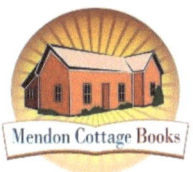

JD-Biz Publishing

Download Free Books!
http://MendonCottageBooks.com

All Rights Reserved.

No part of this publication may be reproduced in any form or by any means, including scanning, photocopying, or otherwise without prior written permission from JD-Biz Corp Copyright © 2015
All Images Licensed by Fotolia and 123RF

Disclaimer

The information is this book is provided for informational purposes only. It is not intended to be used and medical advice or a substitute for proper medical treatment by a qualified health care provider. The information is believed to be accurate as presented based on research by the author.

The contents have not been evaluated by the U.S. Food and Drug Administration or any other Government or Health Organization and the contents in this book are not to be used to treat cure or prevent disease.

The author or publisher are not responsible for the use or safety of any diet, procedure or treatment mentioned in this book. The author or publisher is not responsible for errors or omissions that may exist.

Warning

The Book is for informational purposes only and before taking on any diet, treatment or medical procedure it is recommended to consult with your primary care provider.

Our books are available at

1. Amazon.com
2. Barnes and Noble
3. Itunes
4. Kobo
5. Smashwords
6. Google Play Books

Table of Contents

Paleo Diet – An Introduction

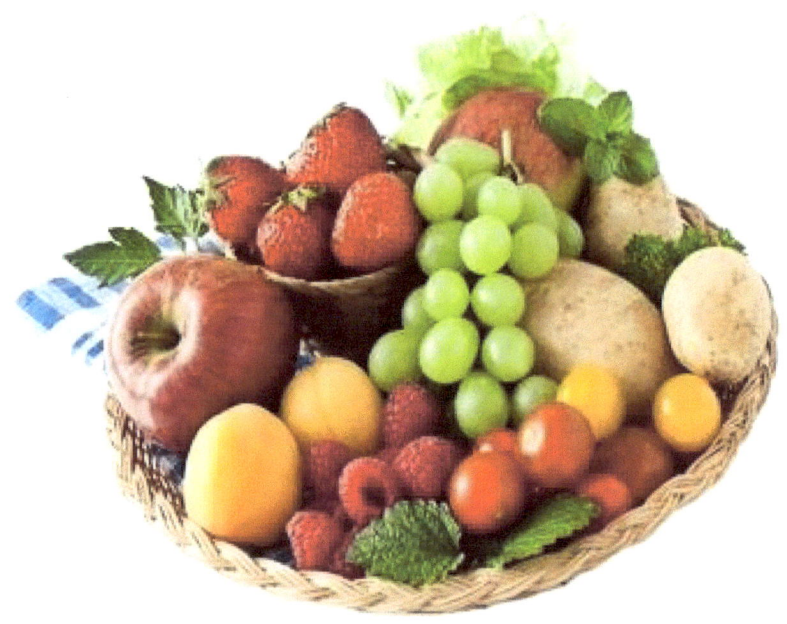

Paleo diet is what our ancestors used to eat tens of thousands of years ago when there weren't any supermarkets or fast-food chains; all they could rely on were their limbs for hunting and edible plants, to fulfill their needs. The Paleo Diet is a restrictive diet; its menu ranges from meat, vegetables and fish to fruits, nuts and sometimes even roots. A detailed table of what and what not, is provided below.

Allowed	Not Allowed
Lean red meats, game meats and organ meats	Grains (cereals such as barley, corn, oats, rice, rye and wheat)
Pork	Beans
Poultry	Legumes
Fish and Shellfish	Dairy products
Eggs	Salt
Leafy and cruciferous vegetables	Refined sugar
Root vegies	Refined fats
Mushrooms	Canned or processed meat
Fruits	Fatty meats
Nuts	Bacon
Raw Honey	Soda and fruit juices
Coconut palm sugar	

This diet was brought into the lime light during the 1970s. Nowadays, it is receiving a lot attention from the public and many even consider it to be the best thing that ever happened to them. It is receiving an equal amount of attention from researchers and dietitians.

How does the Paleo diet attract such a large audience?

It accomplishes this goal by luring people in by the following ways:

- Speedy loss in initial weight
- Illusion of greater control over blood sugar
- Short-termed health benefits by eliminating processed foods from one's diet

But these seemingly amazing, initial benefits come at cost: The Paleo regimen may give you the illusion that it's working, and to some extent that is true but at the same time it would be giving birth to numerous diseases; and that's not all, a lot of mostly harmless yet extremely annoying side effects have also been linked to followers of the Paleo diet. Paleo Diet is also not the most economically viable option when it comes to eating. Meat products have a lion's share in a typical Paleo diet plan and as you all know, meat isn't the cheapest food item out there.

The Trouble Begins

Chapter # 1: Warning Shots

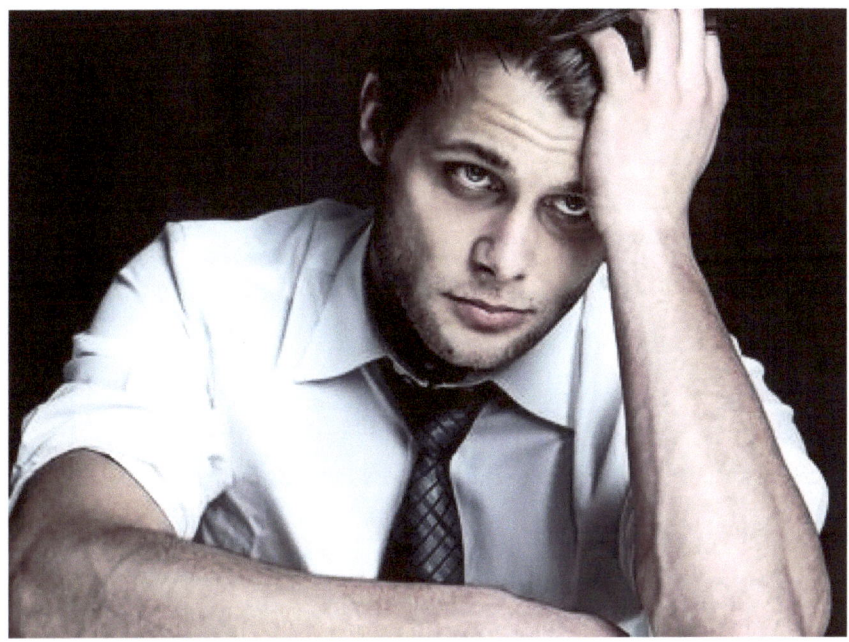

As obvious, the Paleo diet cuts off a lot of carbohydrates and dairy products from one's diet. When you start up with the Paleo diet, the first few weeks might be particularly hard on you. Many Paleo gurus brush this off by stating this as an adaption phase for your body, from a high-carb diet to a low one. Many people fall for this trap and continue with the diet plan but the reality is somewhat different; you will find out soon enough. The following are a list of side affects you may experience when starting out with the Paleo regimen:

- Headache
- Fatigue
- Nausea
- Lack of energy
- Lack of concentration
- Weakness
- Light-headedness
- Dizziness
- Irritability
- Constipation and/or diarrhea
- Body aches
- Cold sweats

You might start experiencing them within the first 12 hours of dieting. These side effects may resolve within a few days or may last for up to 2 – 4 weeks in some extreme cases.

Chapter # 2: Behind the Scenes

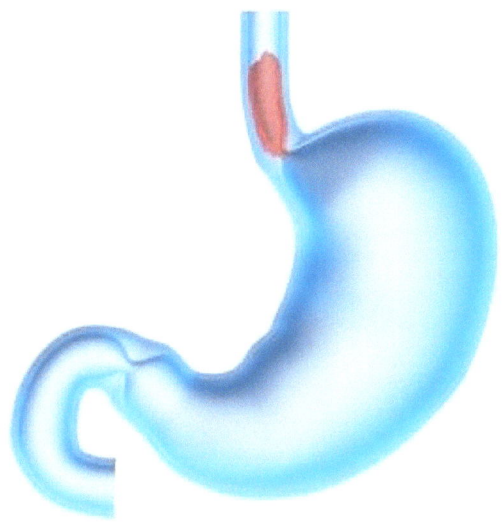

A low carb diet is one in which your body gets less than 50g of carbohydrates a day. When you switch to a low carb diet your body will be in *ketosis*. Ketosis involves your body switching from a carb-burner to a fat one; it means that your body will start burning fat, which you eat and that is already stored in your body, and it's by products for energy. A diet is considered ketogenic when it is very low on carbohydrates. The table on the following page compares different diets and their ketone levels.

During ketosis, a lot of the illnesses stated in the previous chapter will surface. It is told that your body is making a transition from carb to fat for fuel, but the fact is that there is no such thing: You can't "train" your body to use fat for fuel; it is an extreme measure it takes during starvation and lack of food. Changing carbs with fats as the basic source of energy is not viable because metabolism of fats require more energy as compared to the metabolism of carbs.

Type of Diet	Ketone levels
Normal diet	About 0.5 mM
Paleo diet	0.5-3 mM
Ketosis	3-5 mM
Diabetic emergency	15-25 mM

Most of the symptoms stated in the previous chapter are due to severe lack of energy producing foods: carbohydrates. And when these symptoms end, this doesn't mean our body has adapted now; it means that your metabolism has slowed down to allow the transformation of fat into sugar. The transfusion of fat into fuel is difficult job for the body and so this task is only reserved for extreme cases such as starvation as stated above. Once the metabolism slows down to facilitate this process, your energy returns and you begin to feel good again, but this is not permanent. How long a person can run on his/her stored body fat varies from person to person; it could be days, weeks or months depending on the amount of stored fat and persistence your body has.

A very elaborate example of this is working out: physical workout at a slower pace results in the body burning a greater amount of fat and less carbohydrates; this is because the body has time to convert fat into fuel and use it for energy. The reverse happens during high intensity exercises:

Because your body needs an instant supply of energy, it burns carbs as no conversion is required.

Therefore, you don't train your body into doing anything. The body goes at its own pace and does what is necessary to provide fuel. But when your body runs out of fat it begins burning other tissues, starting from the most useless ones; this is where the damage begins. This is when you need to stop following the Paleo diet to prevent any further damage to your body. This process might be useful 10,000 years ago when there were no food stocks but in the 21st century this is madness.

"Given these facts, in combination with the strongly plant-based diet of human ancestors, it seems prudent for modern-day humans to remember their long evolutionary heritage as anthropoid primates and heed current recommendations to increase the number and variety of fresh fruit and vegetables in their diets rather than to increase their intakes of domesticated animal fat and protein." <u>*The American Journal of clinical nutrition*</u>

The Paleo diet being low in carbohydrates also has a diuretic effect that results in your body losing extra water. If you lose this water too quickly, you could start experiencing symptoms of dehydration.

Many of us are fully aware of the addictive effect that grains, dairy and sugar have on us. Biologically speaking they have the same effect on our brains as do drugs, but to a lesser extent. As the Paleo diet eliminates these foods from our diet, we can undergo a withdrawal effect for some time. This effect may last a few days or 1-2 weeks depending on how fast your body can learn to live without these substances.

Chapter # 3: How to ease these side effects?

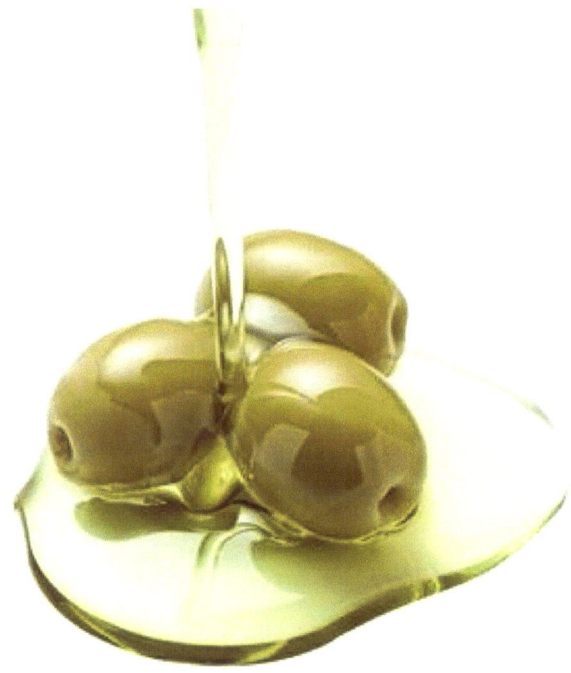

To get these side effects under control while still staying confined within the restrictions the Paleo diet places on you, you'll need to eat more fat: Add 1 - 2 table spoon of coconut oil, extra virgin olive or plants rich in unsaturated fats to your meals. You can also use avocados, olives and nut instead if you don't have easy excess to these oils.

Many people on the Paleo diet practice intermittent faster and skipping meals; this isn't the best option for you, especially if you have issues with your blood sugar, so make sure you ingest at regular intervals. Also, drink enough water to tackle the mild dehydration effect that a low-carb diet has.

You can also add more salt to your food than the Paleo diet if your body is dehydrating too quickly. It's better safe than sorry.

If you work out a lot, you might experience fatigue and weakness during the first two weeks; it would be best to lay off the high-intensity cardio to prevent these symptoms from getting worse.

If your gallbladder was removed, make sure to slowly increase your fat intake when starting out on the Paleo diet; this will help your body adjust by secreting adequate amounts of digestive enzymes. Furthermore, if you are on some kind of medication, it would be best to consult with your doctor first before going through with the plan.

Side effects that play along

Many of the side effects stated in the previous section last only for a few weeks, but there are some that go along as you follow the Paleo diet. There are also side effects other than those stated in the previous section that carry the risk of being long termed.

Chapter # 4: Weakness and Memory Loss

Psychology professor Paul E. Gold has researched the stability of glucose levels in the brain. Working with Ewan C. McNay , they found that as rats went through a maze, concentrations of glucose declined in the animals' hippocampus , a key brain area involved in learning and memory – even more dramatically so in older brains.

Except under conditions of starvation, it was thought that the brain always had an ample supply of glucose. "While this is the case in terms of consciousness, the new findings suggest that glucose is not always present in ample amounts to optimally support learning and memory functions," said Gold, who is director of the Medical Scholars Program in the University Of Illinois College Of Medicine.   "The brain runs on glucose. Young rats can do a pretty good job of supplying all the glucose that a particular area of the brain needs until the task becomes difficult," explained McNay, a postdoctoral researcher in psychology at Yale University. "For an old rat given the same task, the brain glucose supply vanishes out the window. This correlates with a big deficit in performance. A lack of fuel affects the ability to think and remember."

-Study conducted by Professors Paul E. Gold and Ewan C. Mcnay

Brain cells require twice the energy than any other cell in the human body. For most of us even thinking can be a tiring process, even exhausting in a few cases. Research has shown that mental concentration drains glucose from a part of the brain associated with memory and learning.

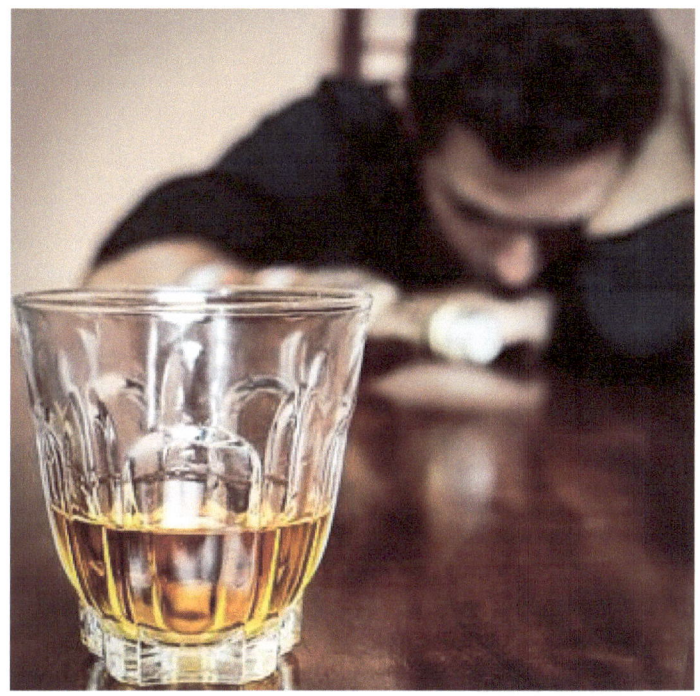

A diet consisting of grains and legumes is mostly eaten because there are a large amount of carbohydrates in them. As the Paleo diet restricts from consuming carbohydrates, your body is forced to switch from carbs to fat for fuel; fat and proteins are first converted to carbohydrates which are in turn converted to glucose. Unfortunately this is not how your brain works. Your brain does not have any stored supplies of fuel; it requires a constant supply from the bloodstream. The conversion process takes too long and as a result your body experiences symptoms like fatigue, trembling and lethargy. In simple terms, the rate of supply of carbs to the brain takes a huge hit when you switch to the Paleo Diet resulting in brain dysfunction.

Furthermore, glucose is extremely important to improve and maintain your memory. As it is the only primary source of energy it is rapidly used up during mental activities such as memorizing. As the blood glucose level drops one finds it extremely hard to stay attentive, process auditory and visual information.

When Dr. Carol Greenwood tested the memory of older adults after they ate a breakfast of mashed potatoes or barley, she found that "eating carbohydrate foods can improve memory within an hour after ingestion in healthy elderly people with relatively poor memories."
In another study, Greenwood and her colleagues at the University of Toronto gave a group of healthy senior citizens a bowl of cereal and milk, along with white grape juice for breakfast. Another group only drank water. When tested twenty minutes later, the cereal-eaters had a better memory – able to remember 25% more facts.
Not only does a diet lacking in carbohydrates cut off the brain's main energy supply, Greenwood said a scarcity of glucose can impede the synthesis of acetylcholine, one of the brain's key neurotransmitters.

-Study conducted by Dr. Carol Greenwood

Chapter #5: The threat of Hypothyroidism

This is as frightening as it sounds. Most of us switch to Paleo diet for weight loss but if you undergo this condition, you'll watch your bathroom scales go in the forward direction. And that's just one of the problems which you will have to deal with.

Glucose is required at a constant rate to convert T4 into T3 (active form of thyroid). Since the Paleo diet lacks in adequate amount of carbohydrates, your body goes into starvation mode. The thyroid gland attempts to regulate your body's energy by lowering the metabolic rate resulting in a lower amount of T3 being produced. This is hypothyroidism. The table below gives the normal and abnormal levels of the thyroid hormone:

	Normal	Abnormal
T4	4.11 ug/dl	More or Less than the normal value
T3	110-230 ng/dl	More than the normal value

Hypothyroidism results in an upset in the normal balance of chemical reactions in your body. The symptoms are not noticeable in the early stages, but overtime, untreated hypothyroidism can result in numerous health problems. Some of the signs and symptoms are listed below:

- Increases sensitivity to cold
- Dry skin
- Constipation
- Dry skin

- Weight gain
- Puffy face
- Hoarseness
- Muscle Weakness
- Elevated blood cholesterol level
- Pain, stiffness and swelling of joints
- Thinning of hair
- Slowed heart rate

This condition can be controlled to some extent by increasing the intake of vegetables, mostly those prescribed in the diet.

If you think you are undergoing hypothyroidism do not panic as very accurate thyroid function tests to check for hypothyroidism are available nowadays. You should consult your doctor and if you are lacking a thyroid hormone, a synthetic dose can be given to you.

The Paleo diet is also not a good idea for teens because hypothyroidism in them can lead to:

- Poor growth, resulting in short stature
- Delayer development of permanent teeth
- Delayed puberty
- Poor mental development

So think twice before switching your family to the Paleo diet.

Chapter # 6: Vitamin B-Complex Deficiency

B-Complex is a synergy of 8 different vitamins, enzymes and minerals. Their names and abundance in Paleo food sources is shown in the table below.

	Name	Also known as	Provided by the Paleo Diet
1.	Vitamin B1	Thiamine	Yes
2.	Vitamin B2	Riboflavin	Partially
3.	Vitamin B3	Niacin	Yes
4.	Vitamin B5	Panthotenic acid	No
5.	Vitamin B6	Pyridoxine	Yes
6.	Vitamin B7	Biotin	No
7.	Folic acid	-	Yes
8.	Vitamin B12	-	Yes

The Paleo diet is good enough in providing most of the vitamins and nutrients but this does not mean that there is no longer a need for other vitamins. All of these vitamins are required in conjunction to form the B-complex, therefore if one goes missing the whole structure crumbles. The following are summaries on those vitamins that the Paleo diet fails to provide:

1. Vitamin B2:

This vitamin is required to protect cells from oxygen damage. Like the other minerals and vitamins that form the B-complex, this vitamin plays a key role in energy metabolism and for the metabolism of proteins, fats, ketone bodies and carbohydrates. Moreover, it keeps the saliva lining in the mouth healthy. The most common sources of this vitamin are dairy products, legumes and leafy green vegetables. The Paleo diet excludes dairy and legumes in its diet plan so it is highly probable you'll run low on this vitamin if you don't eat enough green vegies. If you do you'll face mouth inflammation, particularly of the area surrounding the lips; and your tongue will become sore.

2. Vitamin B5:

This vitamin is needed to release energy from fats and sugars. It also supports your adrenal glands which are responsible for secreting hormones that are essential for life, health and vitality. High amounts of this vitamin are found in whole-grain cereals, eggs, legumes and royal jelly. Deficiency in vitamin B5 can lead to sensations of weakness, fatigue and burning foot syndrome.

3. Vitamin B7:

It is necessary for proper cell growth, production of fatty acids and the metabolism of fats. It is also helpful in maintaining blood sugar levels and strengthening nails and hair. Egg yolk and liver are particularly abundant in B7. Deficiency leads to hair loss, inflammation of the skin, depression and lethargy.

To sum it up, deficiency in the B-complex leads to:

- Mouth Inflammation

- Sore tongue
- Fatigue
- Burning foot syndrome
- Numbness
- Tingling
- Heart beat irregularities
- Restless legs
- Memory Loss
- Weakness
- Insomnia
- Depression
- Hair
- Anxiety
- Paranoia

You would need to consume dairy products and eat meals high in unrefined grains including brown rice, wheat, barley, oats and bran, to counter these symptoms. You should consult your doctor if the problem persists.

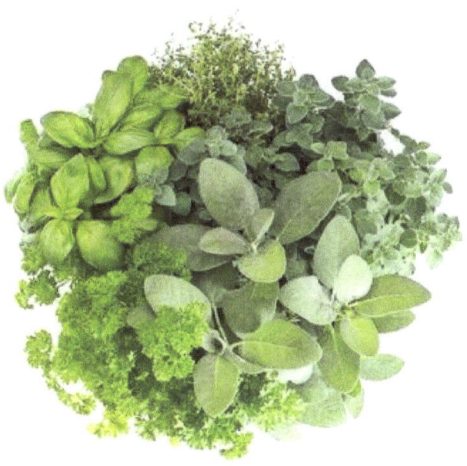

Chapter # 7: Calcium Deficiency

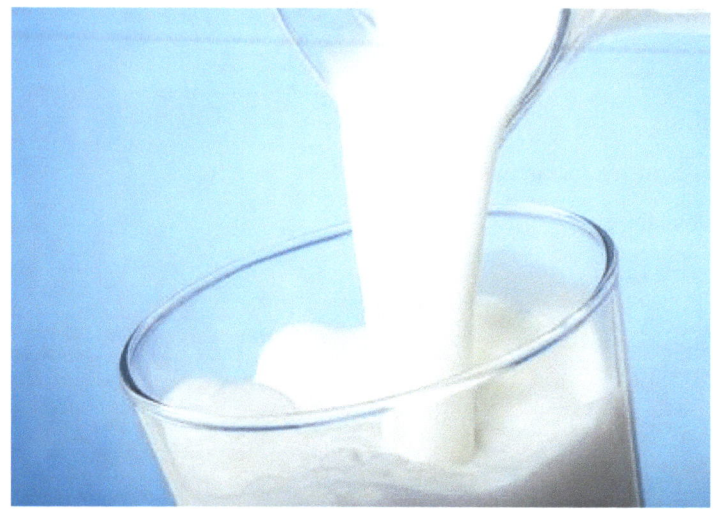

Calcium is the most abundant mineral in our body. 1.5% of our body weight consists of calcium. 99% of this calcium combines with phosphorus to form calcium phosphate which is the hard, dense material our bones and teeth are made of. The remaining is utilized in vital processes in our muscles, blood and tissues. Therefore, calcium plays a very important role in maintaining the strength of our bones. Other benefits and functions of calcium are listed in the table shown below:

	Functions and Benefits of Calcium
1.	Major Component of bones, muscle, teeth and cartilage therefore vital for their growth
2.	Slows rate of bone loss
3.	Slows tooth loss in older people

4.	Prevents Jaw bone from losing its grip on teeth
5.	Helps prevent gingivitis in children
6.	Needed for muscle contractions and relaxations; prevents muscle cramps
7.	Plays a vital role in transmission of nerve impulses
8.	Helps regulate passage of nutrients through cell wall
9.	Needed for normal heartbeat
10.	Needed for blood vessel expansion and contraction; helps regulate blood pressure
11.	Helps blood to clot properly
12.	Reduces the risk of colon cancer
13.	Responsible for the activation of several enzyme systems needed for biochemical processes
14	Calcium helps in alleviating insomnia

Apart from the functions and benefits stated above, calcium holds a vital place in the day to day lives of women. Calcium deficiency may result in a change in menstrual flow. Furthermore, calcium plays a very important role in the development and growth of the fetus during pregnancy. According to a report published in the medical journal "Therapeutische Umschau", the fetus requires between 50 and 300 mg of calcium for proper growth. It has been proved that calcium supplementation reduced the danger of preeclampsia; a hypertensive condition which can lead to pre-mature birth of the baby and in severe cases even lead to abortion. Moreover, mothers lacking appropriate amount of calcium in their bodies tend to deliver babies with low bone-mineral density. Simply put, bone growth is retarded in these babies. Therefore, it is absolutely vital for mothers to eat foods high on calcium.

Foods high on calcium include:

- Milk
- Buttermilk
- Mozzarella Cheese
- Whey
- Yogurt
- Goat's milk
- Collard greens
- Dandelion greens
- Mustard greens
- Spinach
- Turnip greens
- Wing beans

As the Paleo diet does not allow any dairy intake; followers of the regimen are left with only vegetables to boost their calcium reserves. And that's not it; a diet that is high in fat and proteins can decrease calcium up take significantly therefore, Paleo diet followers must eat extra amounts of the vegies stated above to fulfill their calcium needs. Inadequate intake of calcium has no effects in the short term but the situation can get worse in the long term. Symptoms of calcium deficiency are stated below:

- **Osteoporosis:** This is characterized by brittle and porous bones. This happens when the body starts to pull out calcium from bones to provide for other processes. This process is especially speedy in females- especially post-menopausal females.

- **Rickets in children:** Bones become soft and pliable to such an extent that they bend, resulting in skeletal issues including bowed legs, knock-knees, spinal curvature, narrowed chests, bulging forehead and increased joint space.
- **Rickets in adults:** Bones become soft and prone to fractures, limbs and spines deform and arthritic-like pains become common
- Tooth decay.
- Body becomes to more intoxication by lead. This is supported by the fact that children with more teeth cavities have a higher level of lead.
- Brittle nails.
- Risk of high blood pressure
- Insomnia.
- Chronic fatigue.

If you experience these symptoms and if vegetables aren't fulfilling your calcium needs; consult a doctor who will prescribe a calcium supplement of a specific amount to you.

Chapter # 8: Sodium Deficiency

Sodium is another key mineral in the human body. About 55 % of the body's sodium occurs in blood plasma, 40% is contained in our bones and 2-5 % is found in cells. This distorted distribution of sodium is crucial for life. It is needed to regulate blood pressure, passage of nutrients into cells and to ensure that proper nerve conduction. During the day the intestines absorb dietary sodium whereas the kidneys excrete an equal amount into the urine. In case of low sodium consumption the intestines absorb more sodium and the kidneys excrete less.

We acquire most of our sodium from table salt and fresh eggs. Celery and oysters are also known to contain sodium. Followers of the Paleo diet are restricted to oysters and celery, therefore if they don't eat the right amount, they can be facing a lot of problems most notably hyponatremia.

A drop in sodium levels is known as hyponatremia. It can be caused by abnormal consumption of water, consumption of a low salt diet for a long time, excessive exercise that results in sweat and/or by diseases that weaken the body's dexterity to normalize sodium.

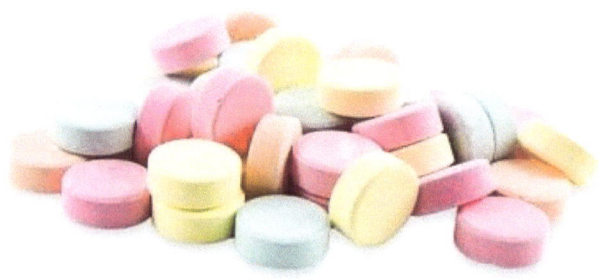

Extreme and prolonged cases of dehydration, due to diarrhea, have been reported to result in hypernatremia. This is simple as diarrhea results in loss of 8-10 liters of fluid containing sodium, water and several other nutrients on a daily basis. Excess of water is one of the other causes of hyponatremia; as the bloodstream absorbs water, this dilutes the sodium in the blood. Beer that is water low on sodium can also be a source of hyponatremia when joined with a poor diet. Studies have shown that 30% of marathon runners undergo mild hypernatremia during a race. Lack of sodium in severe cases can result in strokes. This happens due to increased swelling of the brain's cells resulting in an increase in pressure against the skull. This pressure is commonly taken as a headache but if left untreated can result in a stroke. This further leads to coma and seizures.

Problems linked with hyponatremia include:

- Tiredness
- Headaches
- Muscle cramps
- Disorientation
- Nausea
- Seizures
- Coma
- And if left untreated even death

Hyponatremia can be treated by ingesting water containing 5% sodium. This enters the blood stream and balances the sodium levels. If you feel that your troubles aren't going away, don't hesitate and consult a doctor.

Chapter # 9: Bad Breath

This is the least harmful but most embarrassing side effect of the Paleo diet.

One of the causes is ketosis which was described in the previous section as the process when your body switches to carb to fat for energy. One of the by-products of ketosis is acetone, a certain chemical that has a discrete odor. High levels of acetone production leads to ketogenic breathe. Acetone is released both in your mouth and urine. Its smell is described as those of rotten apples. The severity of this condition is dependent on your height, weight and the amount of carbs you consume daily.

You can make a few additions in your diet to minimize this "keto-breath".

- Start drinking 8 glasses a day.
- Chew mint, parsley, cloves, and cinnamon.
- Chew sugar free gums and mints.

The second cause of bad breath is metabolism of proteins as a result of which ammonia is formed. Meals high in protein result in an increase in the amount of ammonia in breath and urine. Small amounts are not noticeable but the condition can worsen if left untreated. The only solution to this problem is consumption of a higher percentage of fats rather than proteins but this would go against the core principal of the Paleo diet so the choice is yours.

Effects on those with Medical conditions

Chapter # 10: Effects on Type II diabetics

Followers of the Paleo diet claim that it is good at controlling blood sugar levels. But these claims still lack some solid evidence to support them. There are only two plausible explanations to these claims.

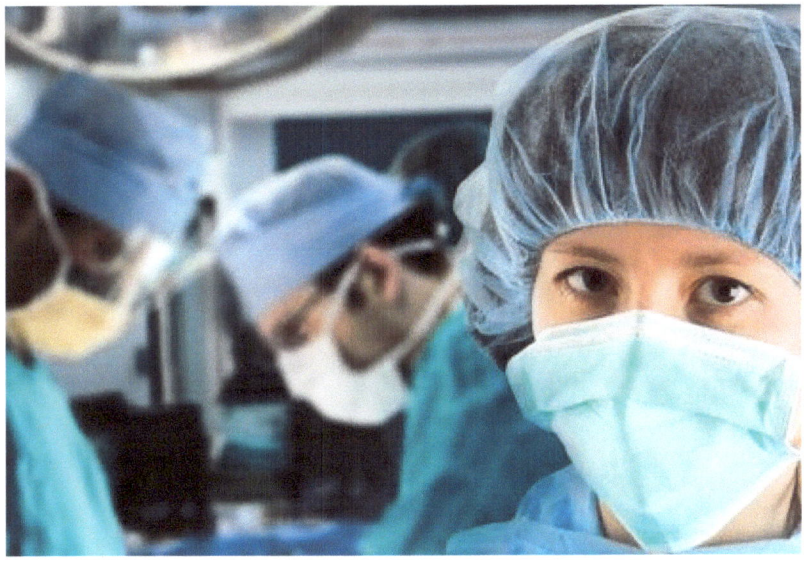

One of them is the loss of weight when one switches to the Paleo diet. Being overweight is the biggest factor in promoting type 2 diabetes. The second is backed by a small study comparing the Paleo and traditional diets and finally measuring blood sugar. Paleo diet performed quite impressively at balancing sugar levels. But this approach still needs to be studied before any long-term conclusions can be drawn. Moreover, diabetes expert still recommend a diet full of whole foods and dairy products to counter diabetes.

Researchers from Yale University studied a group of young adults whose grandparents were diabetic. *Some of these adults already had a resistance to insulin as well as higher levels of intra-myocellular lipids. When these lipids get collected in the cell; glucose is released resulting in high circulating blood glucose levels. The intra-myocellular lipids build up in muscle cells when too much fat is consumed.* Several other studies have also concluded that when a low-fat diet, comprising of whole foods is consumed the intra-myocellular lipids clear out from the cells and the blood sugar level returns to normal. When on the Paleo diet, you will be mostly consuming fat dominant foods. This will result in those lipids building up at a fast rate. To clear out these lipids you will have to start consuming cereals and legumes again.

Furthermore, you can't just quit when on the Paleo diet. Why is that? When you eat a diet high in fats and proteins, your body gets even less able to handle carbohydrates than before. This happens because your intra-myocellular lipids continue to deposit on this high fat diet so now your blood sugar level becomes even more uneven when consuming carbohydrates. Thus, you'll have to slowly retract from the diet until you can finally get rid of it.

Chapter # 11: Effects on Cardiovascular Health

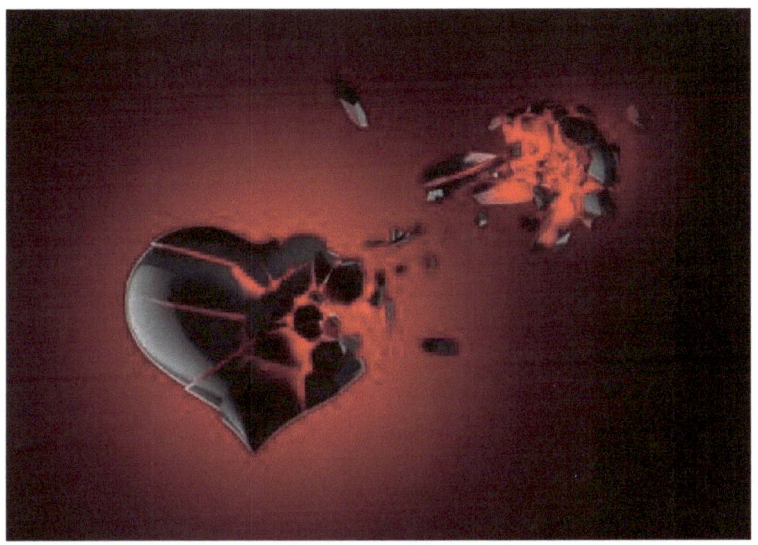

Some studies link the Paleo diet with a reduction in cholesterol, blood pressure and triglycerides, which is a fatty substance responsible for raising risk of heart disease. Studies make the switch from carb to fat as the core reason for their claims. The problem with these studies is their quantity. Studies have been mostly clinical, narrow and had a small test sample; this reduces their credibility. Thus, most experts advise against the protein high Paleo diet when it comes to heart issues.

In a poll conducted to find out the best rated diet among heart experts; Paleo diet was among the least rated diets. No doubt the switch from carb to fat has a positive impact on heart but at the same time a high amount of proteins can limit this beneficial effect. For a better heart you need to limit your diet according to some rules and regulations.

- You should consume **saturated-fat** less than 7% of your daily calories.
- **Trans-fat** should be less than 1 % of your calorie intake.
- Less than 250g of **cholesterol.**

A table of what and what not is given below.

Allowed	Not Allowed
Fresh fruits and vegetables	Coconut
Whole-wheat flour	Vegetables with creamy sauces
Whole-grain bread	Fried vegetables
High-fiber cereal	Canned fruit with heavy syrup
Whole-grains such as brown rice and barley	Frozen fruit with added sugar
Oatmeal	White flour
Ground Flaxseed	White bread
Olive oil	Muffins
Canola oil	Frozen waffles
Margarine-free of Trans-fats	Biscuits, cakes and doughnuts
Low-fat dairy products: skimmed milk, yogurt and cheese	Buttered popcorn
Egg whites	High-fat crackers

Cold water fish such as salmon	Butter
Skinless poultry	Lard
Legumes	Bacon
Soybeans	Gravy
Lean ground meats	Coconut, palm, cottonseed oils
	Full-fat milk
	Organ meats such as liver
	Cold cuts and fried meats
	Hot dogs and sausages
	Bacons

Conclusion

After reading all the side effects associated with the Paleo diet, it would be quite clear that Paleo diet is certainly not the way to go. It involves numerous risks, hazards and if still one decides to "carefully" follow the plan; he/she would still have to do a lot of research before consuming any foods prescribed in the plan. Therefore, it is best to restrict yourself to certain foods and not a specific lifestyle that comes with it good and its fair share of bad.

Author Bio

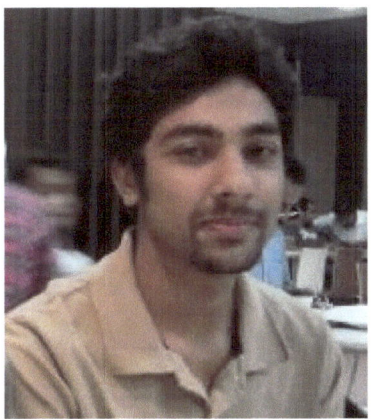

Muhammad Usman is a distinguished medical graduate of Allama iqbal medical college (AIMC). He is a professional writer who has been in the field for more than 4 years. During this time he has produced 10,000+ articles, blogs and eBooks on various niches related to diseases, health, fitness, nutrition and well-being. He is a regular contributor to several journals related to medicine and surgery. He is the editor of several journals and newspapers.

References

1. Walter Voegtlin: The Stone age diet based on in-depth study of Human ecology and diet of man (1975) – CHAPTER 15: A 20th Century Stone age diet (http://www.mitodascalorias.com/wp-content/uploads/2013/06/Voegtlin_1975_The_Stone_Age_Diet.pdf)

2. Wikipedia's definition of Paleolithic diet (http://en.wikipedia.org/wiki/Paleolithic_diet)

3. Walter Voegtlin: The Stone age diet based on in-depth study of Human ecology and diet of man (1975) (http://www.mitodascalorias.com/wp-content/uploads/2013/06/Voegtlin_1975_The_Stone_Age_Diet.pdf)

4. Boyd Eaton, Loren Cordain, Staffan Lindeberg: Evolutionary Health Promotions: A consideration of common counterarguments. December, 2001. (http://thepaleodiet.com/wp-content/uploads/2012/04/Counter-Arguments-Paper.pdf)

5. Boyd Eaton: Paleolithic nutrition – A consideration of its nature and current implications 1985 (http://www.ncbi.nlm.nih.gov/pubmed/2981409?dopt=Abstract)

6. Gary Foster et al. A randomized trial of a Low Carbohydrate diet for Obesity. (http://inspire.stat.ucla.edu/unit_15/NEJM2082.pdf)

7. Staffan Lindeberg et al. Apparent absence of stroke and ischaemic heart disease in a traditional Melanesian island: a clinical study in Kitava. (http://onlinelibrary.wiley.com/doi/10.1111/j.1365-2796.1993.tb00986.x/abstract;jsessionid=7F1EEC9B23FCAD9333A2D12078313A4C.d02t01)

8. Loren Cordain and John Friel: The Paleo diet for athletes. (http://www.trainingbible.com/pdf/Paleo_for_Athletes_Cliff_Notes.pdf)

9. Dr. John McDougall: The Starch Solution (http://www.drmcdougall.com/store_starch_solution.html)

10. Dr. Denis Murphy: People, plants and genes – The Story of Crops and Humanity. (http://www.oxfordscholarship.com/view/10.1093/acprof:oso/9780199207145.001.0001/acprof-9780199207145)

11. Katherine Milton: Hunter-gatherer diets – a different perspective (http://ajcn.nutrition.org/content/71/3/665.long)

12. Alexander Strohle et al.: Carbohydrates and the diet-atherosclerosis connection--more between earth and heaven. Comment on the article "The atherogenic potential of dietary carbohydrate". (http://scholar.qsensei.com/content/1321gb http://www.ncbi.nlm.nih.gov/pubmed/16997359)

13. US. News and World Reports 2012 – Best overall diets (http://health.usnews.com/best-diet/best-overall-diets)

Check out some of the other JD-Biz Publishing books

Gardening Series on Amazon

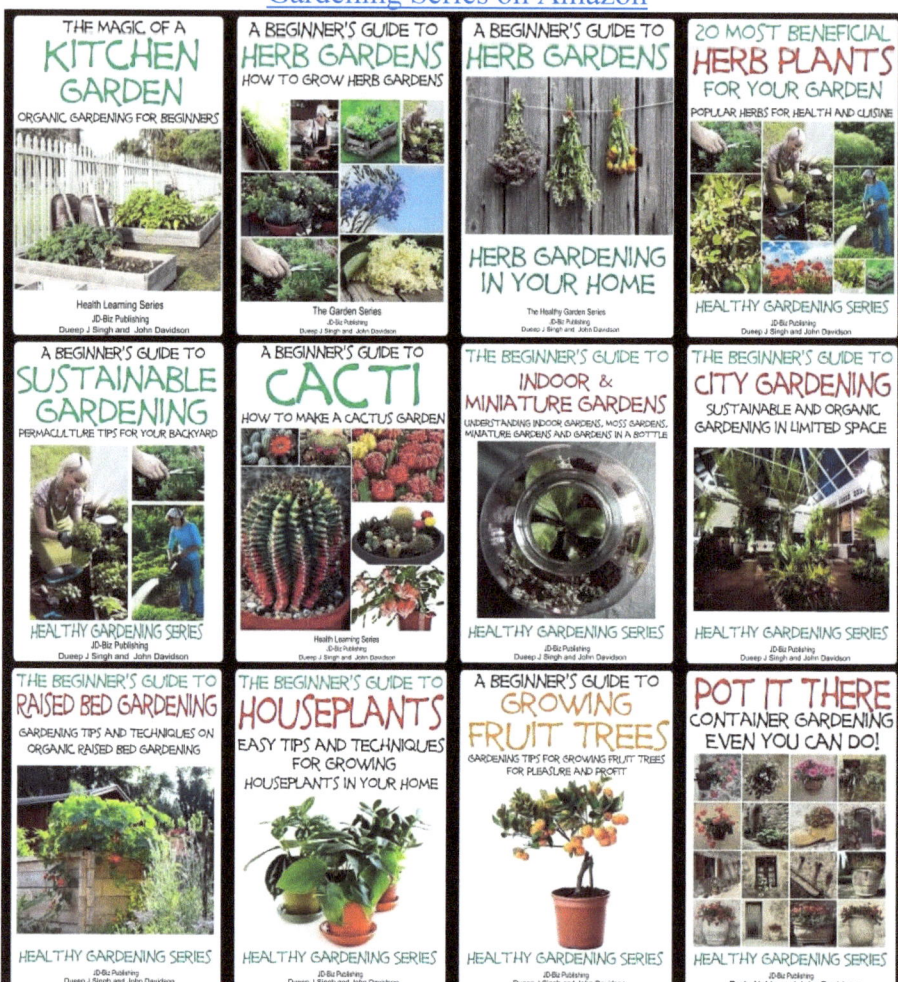

Download Free Books!

http://MendonCottageBooks.com

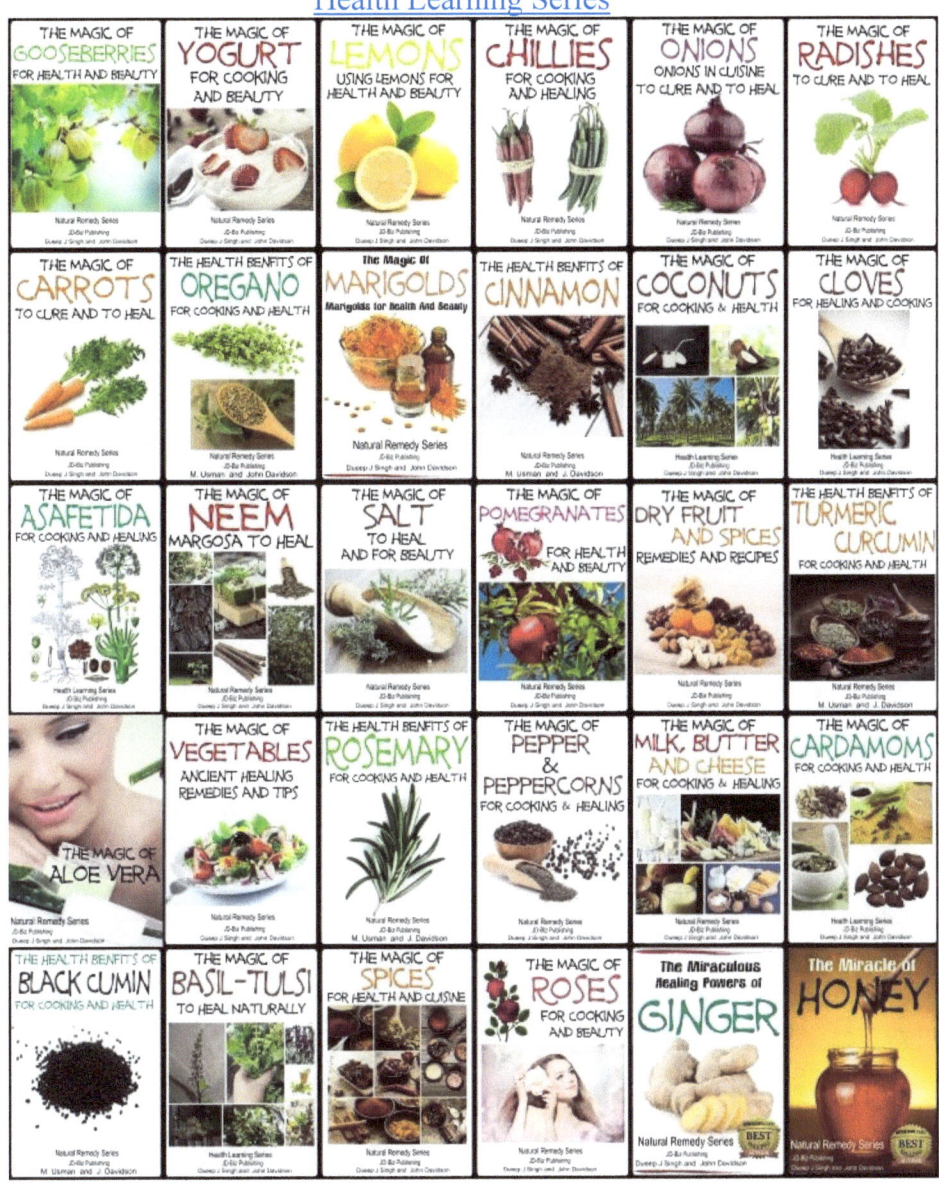

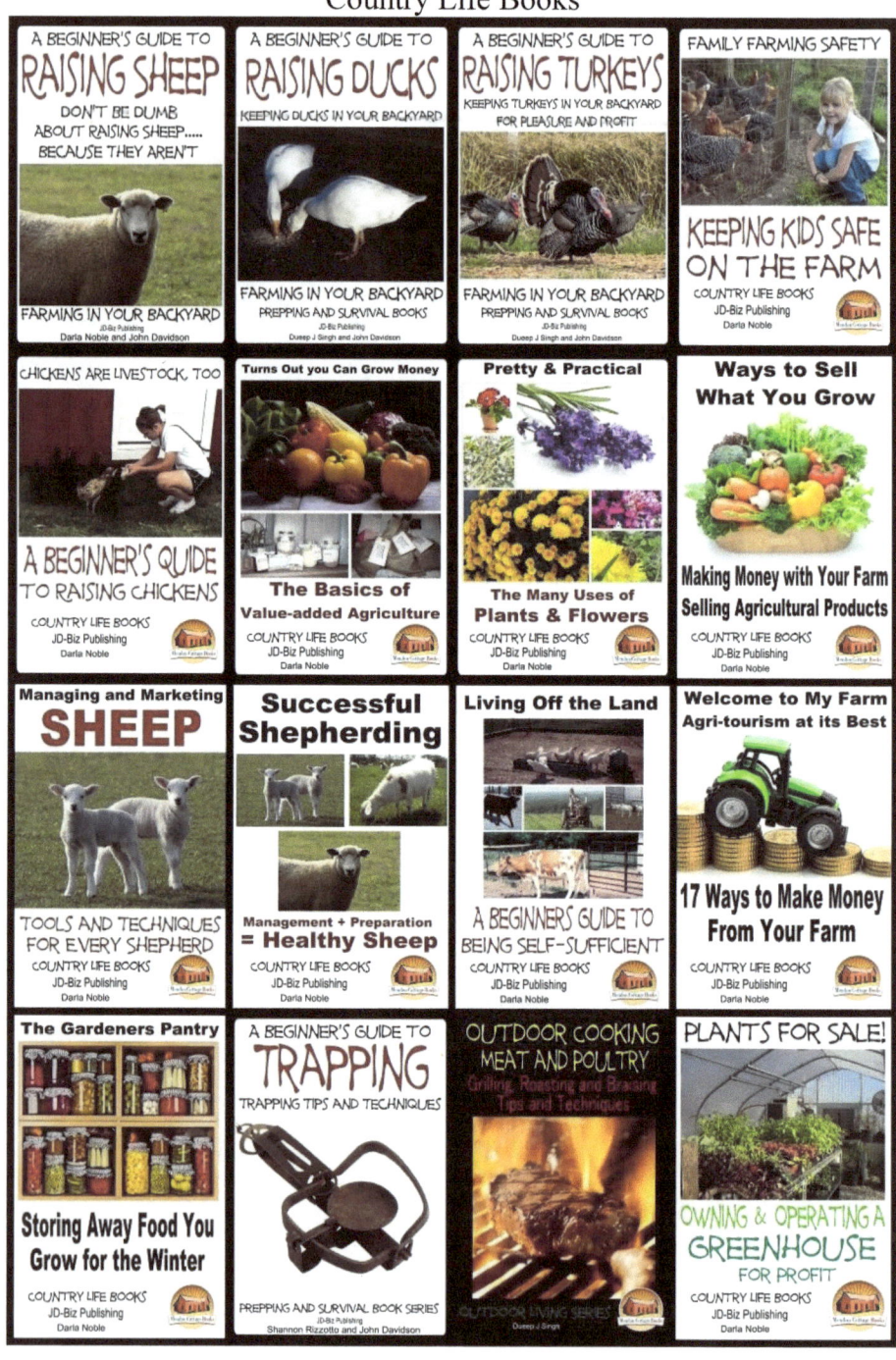

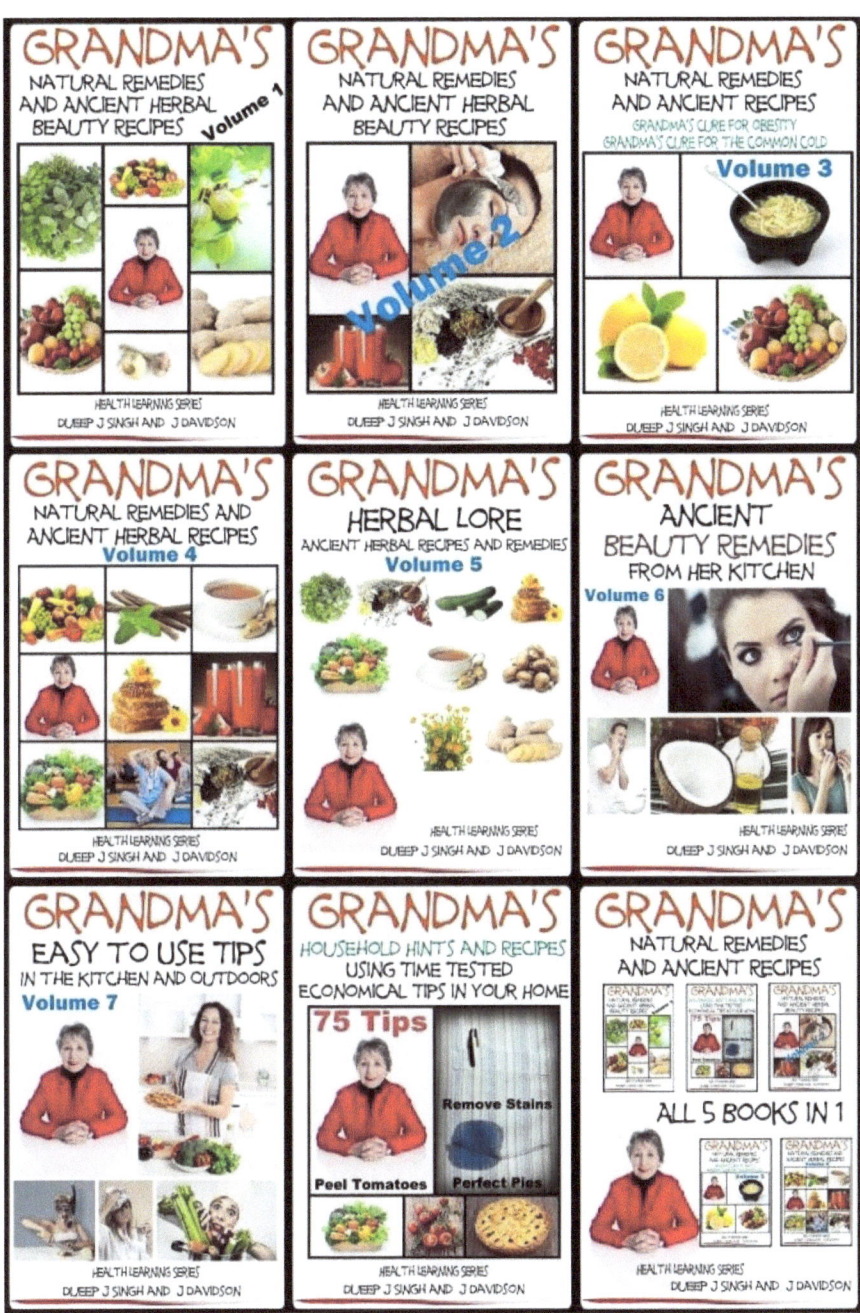

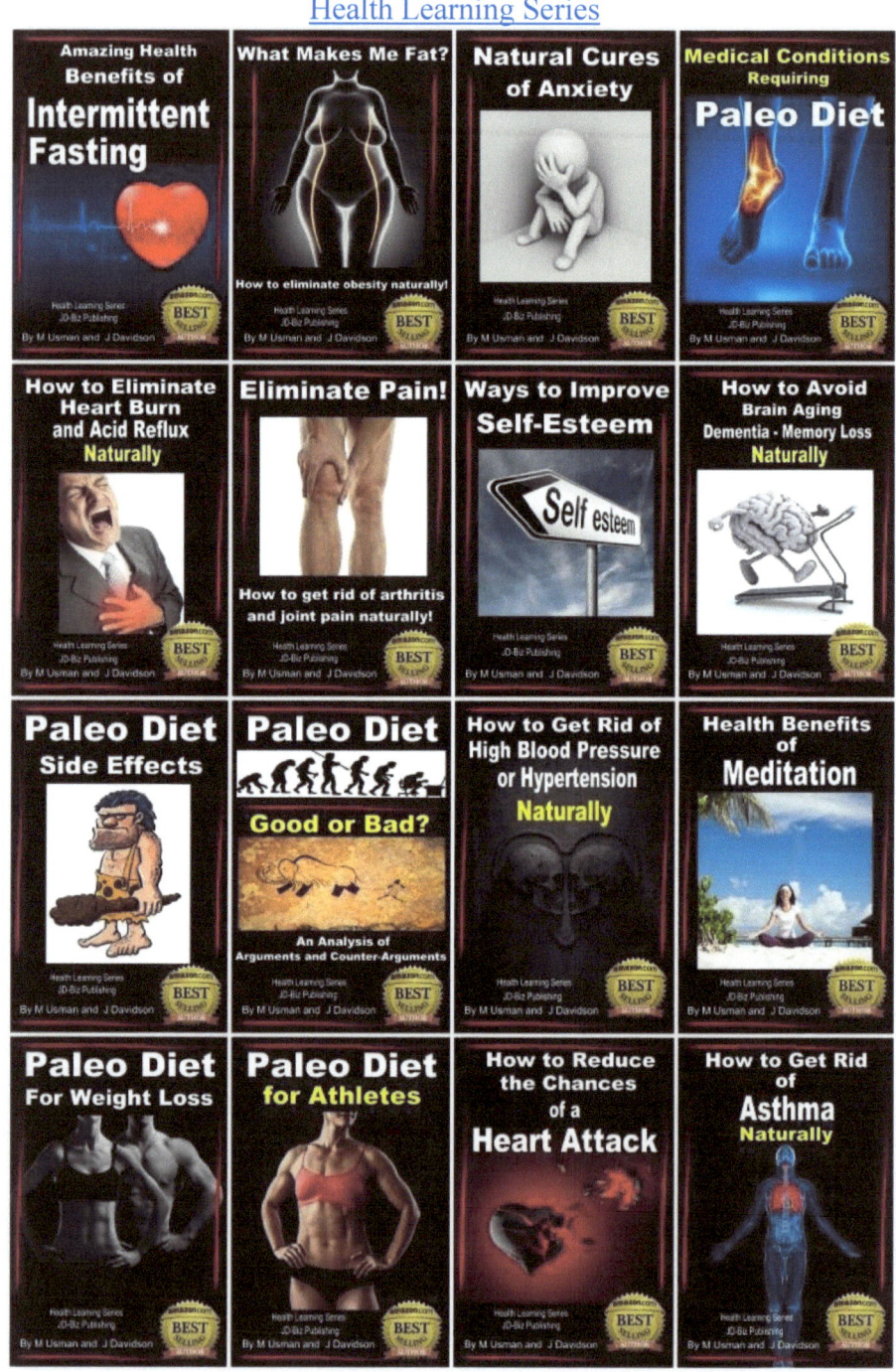

Amazing Animal Book Series

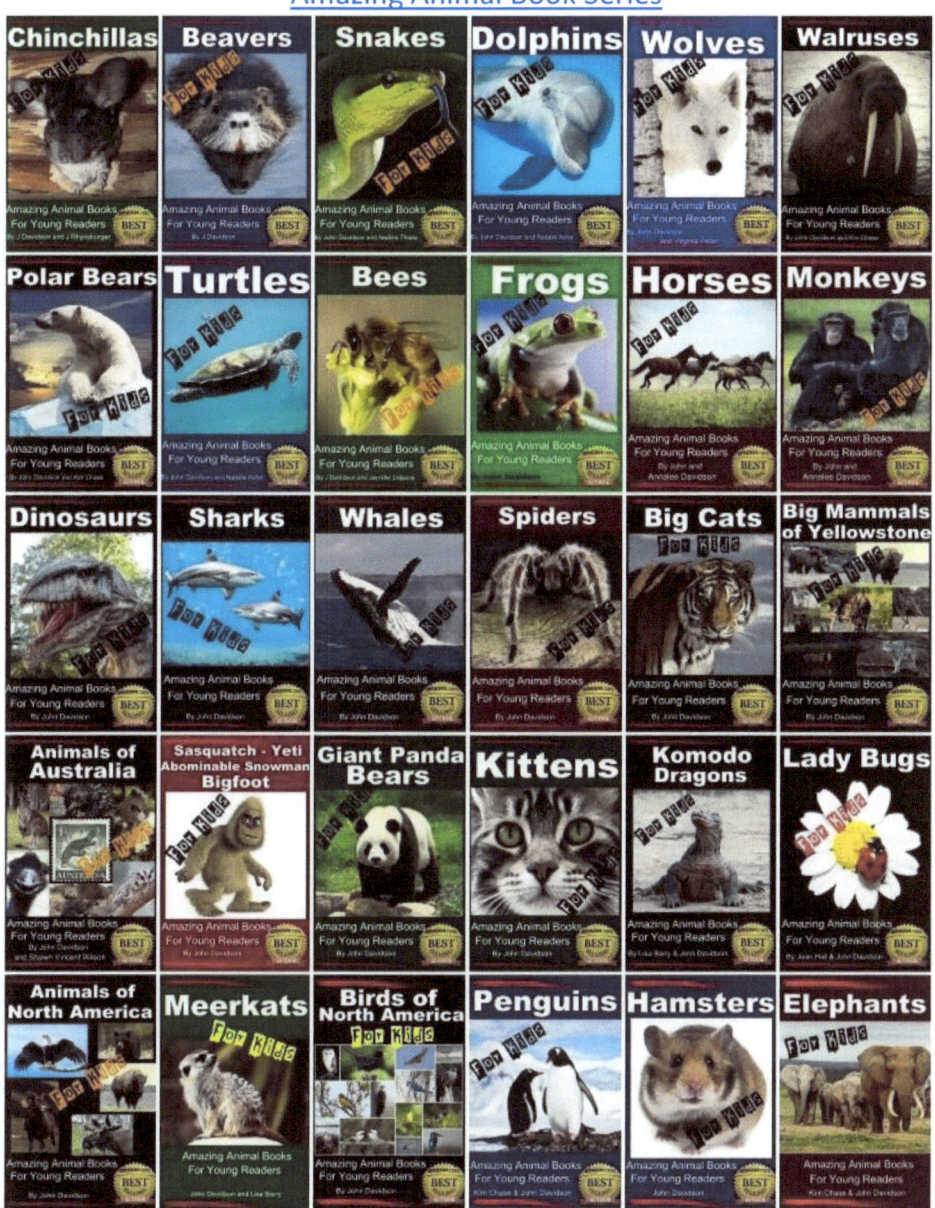

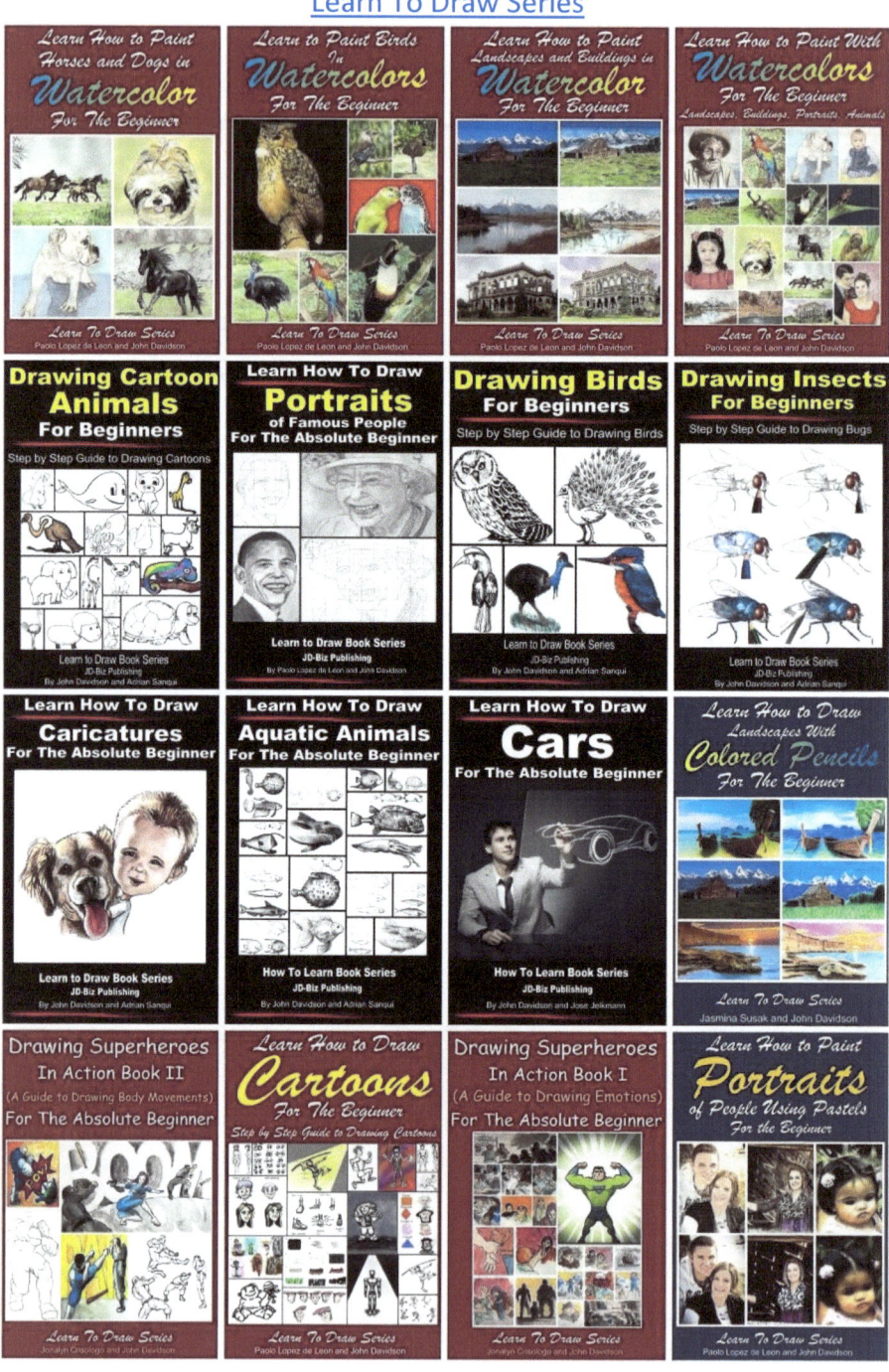

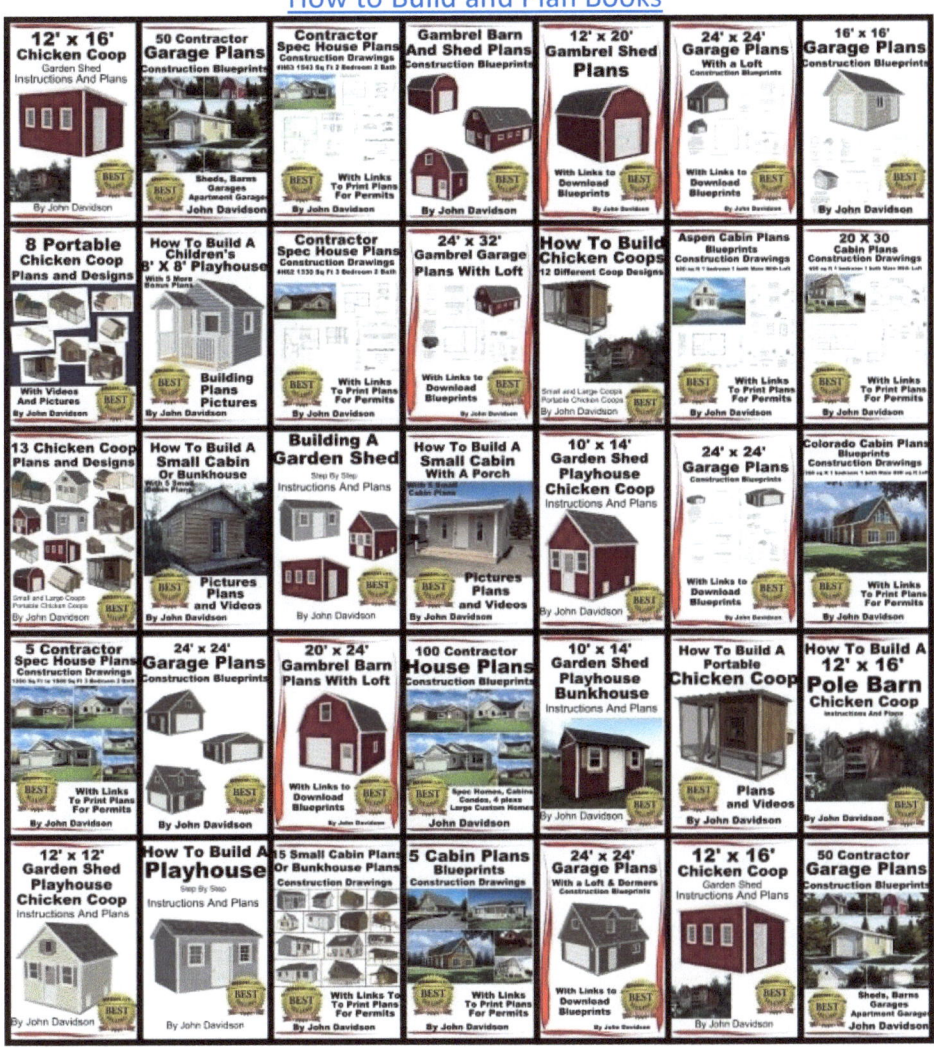

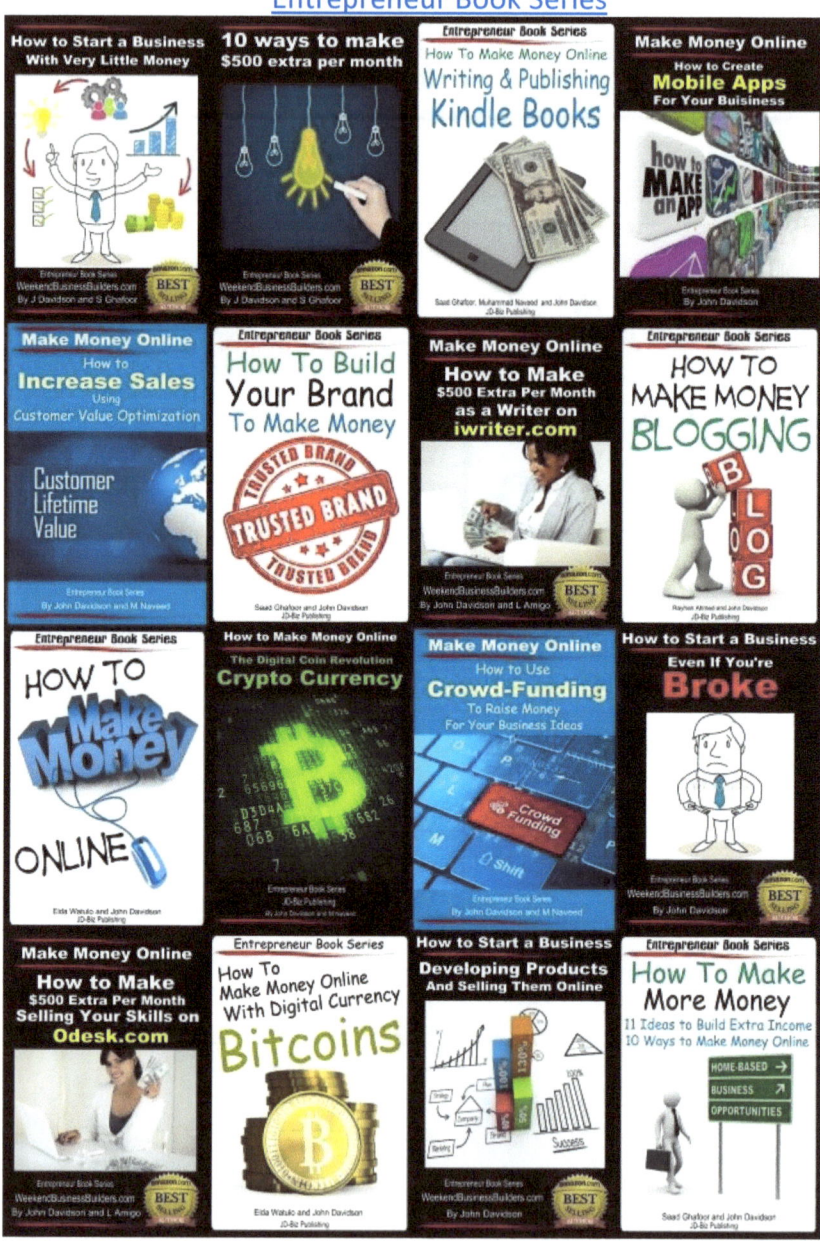

Our books are available at

1. Amazon.com
2. Barnes and Noble
3. Itunes
4. Kobo
5. Smashwords
6. Google Play Books

Download Free Books!
http://MendonCottageBooks.com

Publisher

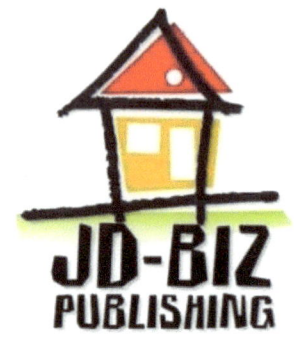

JD-Biz Corp

P O Box 374

Mendon, Utah 84325

http://www.jd-biz.com/

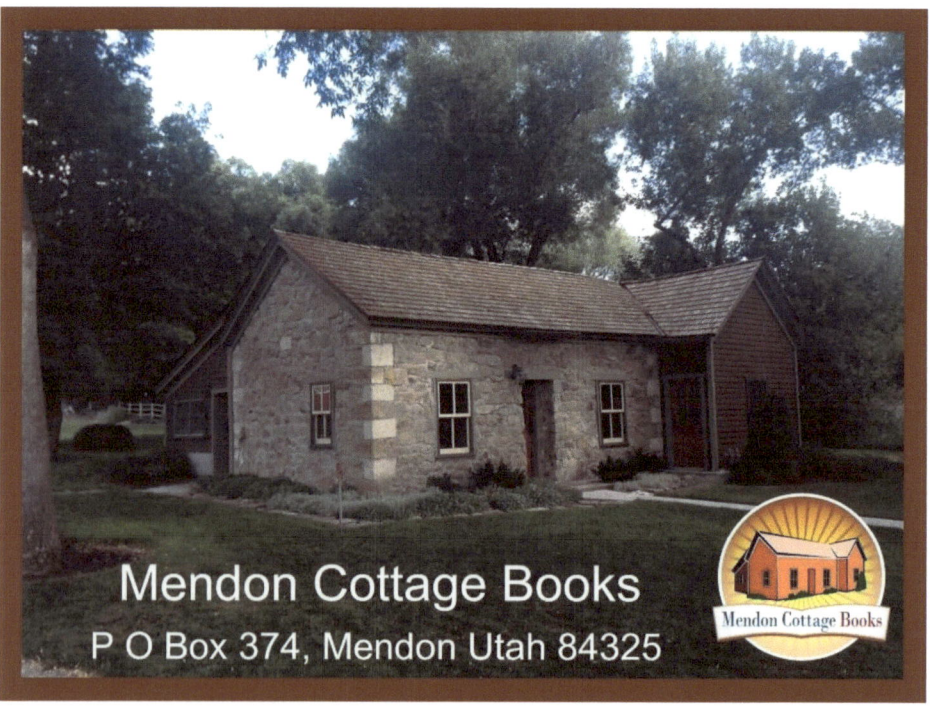

www.ingramcontent.com/pod-product-compliance
Lightning Source LLC
Chambersburg PA
CBHW050836290526
45792CB00001B/410